The Most Important Book You Will Read In Dental School

This book will:

-Prepare you for what may be the most traumatic four years of your life

-Teach you how to get through it with as few scars as possible

-Teach you how dentistry really works outside of school

-Prepare you for **LIFE** after dental school

-Probably offend a lot of dental school faculty

Gregory A. Herman DMD

"Dentistry isn't brain surgery....so don't get so stressed out!"

For Louann and Olivia......I told you I'd eventually get
this thing written!

Table of Contents

Introduction

Congratulations! So you've finished college and decided to do something productive with your life! Something so you don't have to sit in a cubicle/ at a desk for the next forty years worrying if you're going to get fired. Maybe you had an interest in science....maybe you like "working with you hands" *(as we all state on our dental school applications....)*. Maybe you originally planned on going to medical school but realized after a while that there was **NO WAY** you were getting in *(admit it...it's more common than you think)*. Regardless....it doesn't matter. You made a great decision! You won't realize it for quite a few years, but you now have the potential to have an interesting career, help people, be your own boss and have your own business, and make a ton more money than most people. But before you get there, you're going to have to get that dental degree, and that's not easy. This book will help you get there....

"Right, Greg *(I like to go by Greg, not Dr. Herman...like I'm so special)*, but who the heck are you to think that you can teach me better than my esteemed dental school "professors" ?" *(Hint: most of them are just regular dentists like me)*.

Well, by the time you're done reading this little book you'll understand somewhat, but if you follow what I tell you you'll definitely know why once you've been out of school for a few years!

So don't wait any longer....you need to get this information into your brain as soon as possible, preferably before you even apply to dental school.

I want to help everybody though, so I don't want you to feel bad if you are a fourth year dental student and you're flipping through this book and thinking, "Daaaaamn, I wish I could have read this three years ago", or if you are two years into your real world career and hating it *(admit it.....things kinda suck right now)* and you're thinking, "Daaaaamn, I wish I could have read this five years ago".

Nope- unless you're about to retire, this book can still help you. Even if you are established and successful, this book should still help you lower your stress levels by showing you a different point of view. At the very least if you're at that point in your career or even retired, this book will make you laugh as it jogs your memory and you start saying, "Daaaaamn, I wish I could have read this book thirty-five years ago".

Good luck and let's get started!

-Greg

Chapter 1: Before You Even Start

I know this book is called <u>The Most Important Book You Will Read **in** Dental School</u>, but if you're like most dental students, you'll start preparing for dental school before you even get there. That is what this chapter is about, so pay attention if you haven't started dental school yet!

I know you are excited about getting into dental school and the prospects of having a great career and life **BUT**……there is one major thing you need to consider before you even start your "D1 year" :

Dental school is damn expensive!!!!

This one fact can screw up your entire career and even your life if you aren't cognizant of it! It seems that the cost of a dental education can be upwards of $100,000/ year now….and I thought it was expensive when I was in school!

There are three things you can do to mitigate this expense:

1. Go to your state-sponsored dental school

This is really a no brainer. If you have residency in a state that sponsors a dental school, **GO TO THAT**

SCHOOL! You will save yourself thousands of dollars by doing so. Look, you'll learn this as you get through this book, but pretty much all US dental schools are the same. After you graduate you're not trying to get a job as an attorney at a Manhattan law firm. So if you live in New York, go to SUNY Buffalo; don't worry about the "prestige" of Hah-vahd University.

Besides, if you go to school in your home state, you might be able to spend some time at home getting some home cookin' and seeing your family and maybe some friends too. Trust me- the comforts of home will come in handy at times over the next four years.

2) Don't borrow a lot of money

This is and will be huge *(literally)* as you go forward. It's really easy to borrow more money than you need to pay for each year of dental school, because you'll just be filling out paperwork to get the loans and they'll get disbursed to your school to cover costs like tuition and supplies, as well as room and board if you are starting off in a dorm. Nobody will sit down with you to actually show you how much you are borrowing and how interest works and what all this is going to look like in a few years. No....you'll just get a check for whatever you borrowed that goes beyond tuition for you to "live on". It will be a few thousand dollars, maybe more if you need to pay rent, but regardless you'll feel loaded and start the semester and go about your life and forget about the money.

Until.......

1. You're ready to graduate and you realize you spent $25,000 more on your education than it should have costed.

2. You find out you have to start paying these loans back *sooooon*.

3. You learn you can delay payments *(not "not pay" them but rather make proper arrangements to delay paying them)* but realize that like a credit card, interest keeps adding up, and that interest gets **CAPITALIZED** *(tacked onto the principal)* and you end up paying interest on interest, which sucks.....

4. You realize that by the time you are done paying back your loan, because of capitalized interest, you could have paid for someone else to go to dental school with you, which also sucks....

So really try and limit how much money you borrow to go to school. Yes you'll have a decent income when you start working, but life happens and believe me, there are other things like your family, your business, saving for retirement, and all the good things in life that you'll want to spend your money on besides paying back hundreds of thousands of dollars in loans.

Are you still with me? You are? Good.....

So what's the third thing you can do to mitigate the expense of dental school?

3) Join the Military

What's that you say? Join the military?

"But Greg, I want to be a dentist.....not some grunt in the military, dealing with drill instructors and basic training and guns and maybe even fighting in a war.....**WTF**!"

That's right. Join the military. The Army. The Navy. The Air Force. Probably not the Marines as they don't offer to pay for any school anyway, but that's OK because regardless you're probably not cut out for the Marines at this point in your life. Trust me.

This is probably the single biggest regret I've had in becoming a dentist. Let me briefly go over why you should seriously consider joining the military either before or shortly after you get into dental school:

1. **You'll save a ton of money**. If you're lucky they'll cover the whole four years, but at the very least they will contribute a large chunk towards the cost of attending dental school.

2. When you finish dental school you'll have the chance to enter **specialty training** programs through the military. Again, paid for. In fact, you get paid.

3. You'll have the **opportunity to remain in the military as a career or as a reservist**, which I highly recommend. Along with having access to some great military benefits, once you get that twenty years in, there's a nice supplement to your retirement.

Now, I'm not going to go all political or philosophical on you, but chances are you'll eventually feel a **sense of pride** being a part of something bigger than you, being part of our amazing military, and serving your country.

As far as that other stuff about basic training and drill instructors and guns and stuff, you're a dentist and you're not going to be exposed to any "Full Metal Jacket" type of scenarios (*Unless you want to be like my best friend from college who became a lawyer and joined Navy JAG core and felt unfulfilled. He joined the*

*Marines and a did the whole deal and was almost killed multiple times in Iraq. Twenty years later he's still in and he's **AWESOME**.)*

Nope, you're going to go through a short training period at Officer Candidate School- for wimpy, brainy student-types who don't know the first thing about the military *(easy now...I would have been one of them too)*. When you are done you'll be an officer, probably a Second Lieutenant , in the US Military, and people who probably shouldn't have to will have to defer to your "authority".

Then it's back to school... you'll do some more training periodically, then when you graduate you'll have to give some time back to the military for paying for some or all of your $400,000 education. You might get sent somewhere you don't want to go, but they'll work with you and for the most part you'll be doing dentistry all day on a base. Yeah you'll do some military training and drills. You'll probably get deployed somewhere like Afghanistan for six months or a year. Most likely to do.....yep....more dentistry, on soldiers and civilians over there. Sure if the crap hits the fan you might have to pick up a gun and defend something, but I think since all the chaos started since 9/11 only one dentist has been killed while deployed.

In all seriousness....I know it can sound intimidating. It sounds like too much commitment. It sounds a bit.....scary.

But guess what, my young and inexperienced friend? Time goes really fast! Before you know it twenty years will have gone by and you'll be in your mid- to late-forties *(like me)*.

And guess what else? If you follow what you learn in this book……

You won't have worried much about school debt, and because of that you'll probably be fairly rich by now, or well on your way there!

So I urge you, think long-term and consider the military as you enter dental school.

The bottom line is this: unless you are independently wealthy *(in which case why are you going to dental school?)* or you are one of the lucky ones with rich parents who will foot the bill *(yes...you'll meet a few of those)*, go into this knowing that dental school is very expensive, even if you are going to a state-sponsored school. The debt you can accumulate **WILL** be a burden on you, so you will do well to minimize the cost of obtaining your dental degree. Go to a state-sponsored school, borrow as little as possible, and seriously consider joining the military to reduce that cost.

Chapter 2: Starting Dental School

So here you are! You've gotten into dental school....hopefully you are going to a cheaper state school, you're aware of the expenses and debt you're about to incur, and maybe you've even looked into opportunities with the military to help you save money.

On day one of dental school you'll be sitting in some large lecture hall with your class, probably getting all the congratulatory speeches from the administration about how much you've accomplished and how great the next four years are going to be and how awesome your careeer is going to be. Hopefully you won't get the old "Look to your left and right....in four years one of you won't be here" speech *(you'll probably all still be there).*

Don't be fooled.....some of these administrators and instructors will be the bane of your existence over the next four years unless you are great at kissing ass and smiling when you aren't happy! But more on that as we progress through this book.....

The first two years of dental school is mostly bookwork....some science stuff and classes about teeth and dentistry *(I know....surprising, eh?).* You'll take classes like oral pathology, histology, pharmacology, and the big one...gross anatomy *(where you will be dissecting a human cadaver. You knew that, right?)*

You'll take classes like dental anatomy and occlusion *(or how teeth look and work....possibly the driest and* most boring topic you'll ever study), restorative dentistry (or how to do fillings), fixed prosthodontics (commonly known as "caps"), removable prosthodontics (also known to most as "dentures" or "false teeth"), oral surgery (or "pulling teeth"), and endodontics (ie the dreaded "root canal").

(By the way, my use of parentheses above is to introduce you to the idea that a lot of simple things in dentistry are blown out of proportion to make it seem like a bigger, more important deal than it is. I want you to realize this as early as possible because learning to not take things so seriously will make your experience more enjoyable and, as you get used to things and look at them with this frame of mind, even funny!)

Now the thing is, a lot of these classes will make no sense to you, which is normal because you've never been exposed to any of this stuff! And even if you do well in these classes, you won't really understand what you learned until you get to the "clinical" years when you are actually working on patients. And even then, it will seem confusing because very rarely does a patient's actual tooth that you are working on look like it does in a book.

(Here is when those administrators and instructors will start to wear you down....but more on that later in this book. Just know for now not to take what you are studying at this point too seriously...because it's not brain surgery (if you want to feel like it is maybe you should have gone that route or thought about becoming a "researcher" or even ....wait for it...a dental school instructor!) Again, we'll get more into this later).

Now besides briefing you on what you will be doing during the first two years of dental school and giving you a heads up not to take it too seriously, there is still one very important thing to remember:

You still want to try to do as well in these classes as possible!!!!!

Your grades in these classes will be a big part of what determines your class rank and will be really important if you decide you want to specialize down the road. So when you get to the clinic and start working on real people, you can do the best fillings and other work in the whole school, but if you have crappy grades from your first two years, it's going to come back to haunt you.

Remember when you were in high school and you thought, "How the hell is this damn calculus going to help me in the real world???", and in college when you thought, "How the hell is this damn organic chemistry going to help me in the real world???"

You do? Good.

Because in a few years if you want to get into an oral surgery program and you do, you'll be saying, " Ahhh... now I see how that damn histology class helped me!"

(In case you were wondering, histology is looking at slides under a microscope. I know, I know...exciting stuff, but but I hate to tell you won't be doing much of that when you're practicing in a few years…..)

Chapter 3: Feeling Like You'll Actually Be a Dentist One Day!

So now you know just like everyone has told you your whole life, you have to do well and get good grades in dental school too.

"OK I get it, Greg. Sounds a lot like high school and college so far. What about the whole "learning to fix teeth" part?"

Yes yes yes. I will get into that now.....

While you are going through dental school, even though you won't be working on real patients for a while, you are going to be in what when I was in school were called "pre-clinical" courses, or pre-clinic, or pre-clin as most dental students call it.

Here you will be working on an "typodont", which is really just an unimpressive, overpriced dummy head and jaw that attaches to a metal rod at your workstation. *(Remember earlier when I talked to you about how in dentistry they tend to make things sound more important than they are? This is the same thing.)*

Your first use of this dummy will be learning to to do cavity preparations *(ie how to drill teeth)* and restoring the prepared cavity *(ie how to fill teeth)*. Later as you become more versed in the use of the handpiece *(ie the drill)* you will learn how to do crown preparations *(ie how to make teeth peg shaped so fake porcelain teeth will fit over them)*.

Now, here are a few things I to keep in mind while you are in pre-clin:

1. **Working on these dummies is nothing like working on real people**. The teeth cut like butter, there's no saliva, no tongue, the head doesn't move, the lower jaw doesn't close spontaneously, and most importantly, it's not a real person who is afraid something might hurt and doesn't want to be there.

2. You will periodically take "practicals" *(ie tests)* on these things whereby you will prepare the teeth a certain way and **you will be graded on how well you do it the way your instructors want you to do it.**

3. You see the highlighted part of the previous section? Here's the thing....**a lot of what you are taught won't make a lot of sense to you**. And as I said earlier...that's normal; you probably haven't had any exposure to any of this before....it may as well be learning Chinese, right? Right! *(Unless you know Chinese......)*

4. So for now **just follow as best you can what your instructors are trying to teach you** as far as the outcome of what you are trying to do goes. I won't get into specifics, but a lot of what you are doing will rarely be seen in the real world. But if your instructor tells you to take one millimeter off here and one and half millimeters there, for now, just do that and don't worry about why. Because.....

5. Just like I said with all your bookwork classes, **you want to do well and get   good grades in these pre-clinical classes.** These

classes along with those other ones will again, determine your class rank, which as I said before will play a big part in what options you have when as you approach graduation.

One other thing to keep in mind.....your instructors will get to know you in the preclinic. They will know who is doing well on their practical exams and who is sucking. You don't want to be "that student " in their eyes. If you do well, they will think you are awesome and love you and help you; if you suck they will think you are a loser, treat you as such, and make you feel like crap. Remember earlier when I was talking about the first day of dental school and how you will be given inspirational pep talks by administrators and instructors but some of them will be the bane of your existence? Yeah.....

Anyway...on to the next chapter!

Chapter 4: Starting to Work on Real People

So here you are two years into dental school and you are probably itching to start working on real people in the actual dental clinic! You've probably gone down there and observed or maybe even assisted some third and fourth year students already....now **you** want to get going. Besides, by now you probably need something to motivate you and make you realize you are going to get out of this place eventually.

So let's talk about getting into the clinical side of things and working on real live patients...

There are two main things you want to know going into your third and fourth years of dental school and working in the clinic:

1. **This is the part of dental school that will determine how fast you get out by the end of your fourth year.**

   You will have a number of "requirements" to meet to prove your clinical competence, such as so many of such and such restorations, so many dentures, and so many extractions. Basically a well rounded collection of dental procedures. On paper it won't seem like a ton of stuff, but you will be surprised by how difficult it can be to find these procedures on the right patients! When they come along, you want to take advantage, get it done and check it off your list. Make sure you get the credit put into whatever system your school uses too.

You have to be kind of aggressive to get what you need in the clinic. This is why I said earlier that you have to be able to kiss some ass and smile even if you aren't happy! The majority of your instructors will be pompous and will need their egos stroked. Trust me- I saw plenty of instructors who gave the pretty girls all the help they needed, sometimes to the point of doing procedures for them *(I also saw some other behavior that went well beyond what would be considered acceptable or ethical, but as long as you have two consenting adults........),* and there were plenty of instructors who lived vicariously through the "cool guy" students in dental school.

"Are you serious, Greg? We are talking about professional school here, not high school...." Yes, my friend, I am serious. Look, I'm sure this kind of stuff goes on everywhere. I just want you to know it goes on where you are too, so you don't let it distract and discourage you when it rears it's ugly and unfair head.

Usually you could tell these instructors were leading miserable lives or were in mid-life crisis mode. Or you'll realize from looking at them that they have simply always been dorky social losers......

Nevertheless, my point is simply this- get on and stay on their good side and they will help you. If you get on their bad side, or even if they don't really know who you are, they will pay attention to the other students, and those students will get their requirements done faster than you!

One other thing you want to do as you work in the clinic, don't be antisocial..... befriend and take advantage of any relationships you have with fourth year students, as well as your own classmates! They are a great source of patients needing work that you may still need to do, and they can transfer those patients to you if they don't need them anymore. And because they are students like you, they totally understand what you are going through, so the situation is a lot more palatable than dealing with pompous and egotistical instructors who will belittle you and make you feel like scum who could never become a dentist *(more on this later but for now I am reminded of one of my classmates who, upon being chastised excessively by an instructor, simply told him, "I pay a lot of money to go here, but I could go out on the street and be treated like sh*t for free!")*

Are you still with me? Good...remember I said there were two things to know about being in the clinic? So.........

2. Just like in the preclinic, most of what you do in the clinic is not how things are in the real world

I will go into some details about real world clinical work later in this book, because right now technical stuff doesn't matter, and if you are new to dental school and reading this you won't know what the hell I'm talking about anyway!

But for now I want you to understand that what you are experiencing in the dental school clinic with real patients is not how it will be when you are out and practicing. This is a good thing....so as with pre-clinic don't let things discourage you!

1. **Instructors.** As I made clear above, your instructors will be the biggest pains in your a** while you are in school. They won't be there making you feel like an incompetent fool when you are out in the real world practicing!

2. **Equipment.** Chances are when you have a patient to work on in the clinic you will have to set up and clean up your assigned treatment operatory *(there's another fancy word dentists like to use- operatory- like you are performing an operation.....I just call it a treatment room)*. You'll probably have to stand in line at a dispensary to get what you need. Sometimes it takes a while and things get messed up and you'll get blamed and it's frustrating. **This won't happen in the real world.** *(By the way- be nice to the people in the dispensary....they are your friends.)*

3. **Time.** Ahhh time....I wish someone had told me this back when I was in dental school. There are a few things about time that you need to know. First, at least when I was in school, there were only three three-hour appointment slots available: 9 am, 1 pm and 4 pm. So the problem is you will need a three hour appointment to complete a procedure that will take you twenty minutes when you are in the real world because you will be waiting for signatures and getting your work checked as you progress. A signature to start, a signature to give anesthesia, a

signature checking your prep work, a signature checking your restoration, a signature to let the patient leave. It's all to protect the patient of course because you are a student afterall, but it sure does slow things down...

Secondly, because you have so few opportunities to work on patients and when

you do it takes so long, it is hard to get all your clinical procedure requirements quickly. You just can't. So you have to be efficient and make the most of

your time. Choose the right procedure on the right patient. Don't fill a tooth for a basic

requirement that has crazy decay all over the place. If it's a hard procedure like

a root canal, pick an easy case so you can **get it done**!

So now I've covered the bulk of your time in dental school, starting with your early bookwork and taking you through preclinical work and your time working on real patients in the clinic. I'm sure you've picked up some of the themes of dental school if you will *(the so-called "rights of passage")*. Of course a lot of it sucks and is unfair, but if you are aware of it and "play the game", you will get through it. I wish I knew this before I got there and I hope what you have read so far gives you a leg up.

Chapter 5: A Brief Discussion About the Written Board Exams

So while you are dealing with all the stress that your actual dental school puts on you,

you also have to worry about two very important exams that are given not by your school but by the American Dental Association's Board of Examiners, the written national board exams, parts I and II. You will take part I after your second year, and you will take part II during your fourth year. They are multiple choice exams that take a few hours to complete. Basically they test you on everything you have learned in dental school up to that point. Here are the two things you need to know about these exams *(this will probably not surprise you)*:
:

1. THESE EXAMS ARE REALLY IMPORTANT!

2. THESE EXAMS ARE DAMN HARD!

There, are you surprised?

The reason these tests are important is because you can't advance if you don't pass part I, and you can't graduate if you don't pass part II. Now, these aren't licensing exams *(more on that fun later)* but you will need to pass both of these to get licensed once you pass a licensing exam.

Huh??? I know...makes no sense to you right now....board exams....not for the license....licensing exams....need passing board scores to get a license....

Don't worry about it all right now. Just like with everything else, make sure you prepare so you at least pass the board exams. It will be quite a topic among your classmates. There are these things called **dental decks** that are basically flashcards that you can review over and over again. There are **review books** available. You may even get old **copies of previous exams**.....sometimes questions repeat themselves in subsequent years. All of this will hopefully refresh your memory on many topics that you have studied in dental school.

Now, a couple of paragraphs ago I said you want to at least pass the board exams, for obvious reasons. But just like with your classes, your preclinic time, and your clinic time, you will do well to do the absolute best that you can on these exams.

Do you know why? You do? Good. Let me make sure....

Options, options, options! Just like when I said your grades in dental school will determine your class rank and give you more options when you are nearing graduation, so will good board scores. Your board scores help make you comparable to all the fourth year dental students across the country *(and world for that matter)* and play a huge role in whether you get into a residency after you graduate, if you decide you want to apply to any. In fact some states require some postgraduate training, even if it's just general dentistry, to get a license in that state. My state, New York, is like that now.

So just remember, the board exams are important, and they are hard, but you can pass them, and you want to do well on them!

Chapter 6: Licensing Exams

As you approach the end of your fourth year of dental school, you will start to hear a lot both from the school administration and your classmates about whatever regional licensing exam you will be taking. This is the exam that will allow you to apply for a license in the state in which you wish to practice. Unfortunately, for many political and financial reasons, there isn't one exam that covers all fifty states. Heck....some states like Florida have their own exam *(at least they used to)* and they won't accept a passing score from another region. Some states, like Florida again, won't let you simply move there and practice after you have been practicing in Nebraska for twenty years, without taking their exam.

Apparently there are different ways you can fix a tooth in different parts of the United States!

Apparently if you go to one of the best dental schools in the country *(they are pretty much all the same)*, say Tufts or Harvard University, and you settle in Massachusetts to practice for twenty years, you aren't a good enough dentist to just move to Florida and practice there!

Well, I'm sure you know that's not really the case. No, it really comes down to this: Florida is a really nice place to live and practice. And all the dentists living and working down there don't want every other dentist to move there and create more competition. Same goes for places like California (see- I'm not just picking on Florida), though they do offer "reciprocity", or recognize and value your experience and license in another region, after you have been practicing for something like five years.

In addition, these exams are, wait for it.......

DAMN EXPENSIVE!

Again, this is a common theme in the world of dental school and dentistry. There is a lot of money being made by these testing agencies and regional boards. I like to call it a racket, but the bottom line is that whatever area of the country you want to practice in, you are going to have to spend a lot of money for the privilege to do so, **AFTER** you've already paid for or indebted yourself via dental school. This isn't so bad if you are an established practicing dentist with some money to spare......but it sucks if you are a broke dental student!

Soooo....if you are a dental student, you really want to pass any licensing exam you take, the first time you take it. That is what I am going to talk about now.

I know I talked about the expense of these exams above but the first thing you should know about taking

a licensing exam is that they are **very stressful!!!!** You will be finishing up dental school and realize that you won't be able to work in the real world and make money to start paying back your dental school *(and possibly undergrad)* loans, let alone enjoying the fruits of your efforts during school, unless you pass and are able to apply for a license to practice. You may be able to get a temporary license to practice if you are in a residency, but come on....that's not a real license to practice. Some states such as New York may allow you to practice there if you do a residency, in lieu of taking an actual licensing exam. But again, your options will be limited.....you may only be able to practice in that state.

But listen....try not to let these thoughts consume you. You **WILL** pass a licensing exam. Probably the first time you take it. There are, from what I can gather, very few failed dentists out there who finished dental school but could never pass their licensing exam. Failed dentists who lost their licenses because they suck or are stupid-yes, but there aren't many that could never get their licenses in the first place.

So when you get to this point *(and you will)*, stop worrying about passing. You will have enough to worry about just taking and getting through a licensing exam.

So let's talk a little bit about actually taking a licensing exam.....

Now, I only took what was then called the North East Regional Board, or NERB *(a word that still sends shivers down my spine)*. That is because I went to school in Boston which is in the Northeast. Duh....However most of these exam are fairly similar whatever region you are testing for, especially the **paperwork and administrative/ procedural stuff.** So let's start there.

I know you probably think you need to make sure you get the actual procedures done acceptably, and you do, but before you even worry about that, you need to make sure that all the paperwork, even something as simple as putting your name on the forms, is perfect. Even in this modern day and age of computers and online this and online that, you will receive a packet of forms after you sign up for a licensing exam. These are forms that you will take with you to the exam and the examiners will them use to monitor your progress and grade your work. I won't go into specifics about these forms and papers....just make sure your review them thoroughly and fill them out accurately before you get there, as well as when you are there and have to complete them. You will fail if you don't put the patient's blood pressure down, or if you write down the wrong tooth number or surface. **These exams are difficult enough, so don't blow it on something stupid like paperwork**.

Now, as for the exam itself....

There are usually three parts to a clinical licensing exam:

1) **Clinical procedures on a typodont *(the dummy head...remember?)* such as root canal and crown and bridge**

2) **Clinical procedures on a live patient, usually some basic fillings and perio**

3) **A computer-administered written exam**

The first two parts you will probably take either on the same day or on two consecutive days at your testing location. The written part you will sign up for and take another day, within a certain timespan, at a separate testing center.

The single most important thing you need to do during the exam is:

MANAGE YOUR TIME WELL!!!!

None of the procedures you will do on the exam are particularly difficult, especially if you choose your live patients well. More on this later. But all three sections will be difficult if you do not manage your time well.

Now managing your time well probably seems pretty obvious on any exam where you don't have unlimited time to finish, but on these tests you will have a hell of a long time to complete each section and what can happen is you will relax and something will go wrong and the next thing you know you are rushing to finish something and you'll do a crap job on something that should have been a slam dunk.

There's nothing like making an acrylic temporary three unit bridge when you only have a fifteen minutes because the one you have been working on for the last hour cracked when you seated it because it shrunk while it set! Get my point? You do? Good.

Now let's talk a little about the actual exam and how you can make sure you pass it the first time you take it.

First let's talk about the live patient section. Most likely you will be doing a couple of fillings and a quadrant of periodontal scaling *(I didn't mention this procedure earlier but basically if you don't know already, it's a cleaning where you remove tartar build-up below the gumline...again, a complicated name for a simple procedure).*

The filling will be 1) a two surface filling that goes in between two teeth and 2) a one surface filling that goes on the front of a tooth that is usually by the gumline. There are technical classifications and names for these fillings but frankly I don't remember what they are and

I don't want to bore you with unimportant stuff. If you personally care about that, if it makes you feel like a doctor or more professional, that's great....more power to you. But it's really not that important and the people that will one day put money in your pockets won't care either.

Here are the only things you need to know, and it relates to managing your time well:

1. **Get a normal, easy patient that will be easy to work on**. By normal, I mean "not crazy". Make sure they are healthy...no major medical conditions like heart problems! If there are any medical problems, your examiners may not let you even start the procedure. Make sure they will show up for the exam. Make sure they know where to be and when to be there. You may have to get them yourself or somehow arrange for them to get there. You may even have to pay them to incentivize them not to let you down. I know that sounds ridiculous, but it's true, and I want you to pass, so I'm telling you.

2. **Try to find the a case that barely meets the requirements to qualify for the procedure**. If there is too much decay, forget it. If you only need a two surface filling, don't pick someone who needs a three or four surface filling. Look at their x-ray...which you'll need for the exam anyway. Pick a lesion *(the cavity in layman's terms)* that just breaks through the enamel into the dentin *(the layer of tissue under the enamel for you early dental students)*, not one that is blowing through the half the tooth....I guarantee it will be worse when you get into the actual tooth! For the cleaning part, you usually need

six surfaces with tartar on them that can be seen on the x-rays and have gum pockets of a few millimeters. So don't pick someone who has tartar all over the place with deep pockets and bone loss. They will bleed all over the place. It will take longer to get all that tartar off their teeth. If your examiner even lets you start on such a patient, you will still have a better chance of not doing a good enough job and failing.

Next let's talk about the typodont procedures. Usually they are 1) a root canal on an upper front tooth and 2) a three unit bridge preparation and temporary crown and/ or a single crown preparation and temporary crown. Some regions may have some denture stuff but I personally had no experience with that on my exam *(yet apparently after I passed I was ready to make dentures in the real world....)* so I won't discuss that. Just know your denture stuff for part II of the National Board Exam and for the written part of your licensing exam.

Now, here is what you need to know for these procedures for this part of the exam:

1. The root canal exam is pretty easy. You will be given the tooth first to measure the length from the edge to the end of the root. Be very precise and remember this number and get it right! You will then install it on the dummy head and not get another chance to measure it. I won't go into the details of the procedure itself because by the time you are taking this you will know how to do a simple root canal like this *(plus it's damn boring)*. Just make sure your root canal fill matches your measured landmarks from before

you started, follow all the standard procedures, and you will pass with no problem.

2. For the bridge and/ or crown, I'm not going to discuss the tooth preparation as again, by now you should know what you are doing. However, making a nice, passable *temporary* crown or bridge is what will kill you, so here is how you make one. First, before you start, take a good impression of the tooth and/or teeth you will be working on. Use a PVS impression material *(again, for the newbies, don't worry about what this means right now)*. Use a simple automixing temporary material in a cartridge gun. Don't even think of using one old style powder/ liquid systems that you mix yourself *(like I did....probably 5 times before I got it to work....get it?)* Bring your slow speed drill and use Soflex discs, or something similar, to trim up your temporary. You can use acrylic burs to trim away initial bulk and contour, but the soflex discs will let you fine trim the edges and in-between areas without damaging them. They were the key to me making a passable *(it actually came out pretty nice)* temporary. I didn't have them the first time and did not pass the first time because my temporary didn't come out well *(actually it sucked)*.

Finally, there is **the written exam**. I'll keep this really brief. You took and presumably passed Part I and Part II of the National Board Exams. Study and prepare the same way and you will pass. This is easier.

There are a couple of things I want you to keep in mind when you take a licensing exam. I know I said a lot of not so nice things about your dental school instructors and administrators. **AND IT'S ALL TRUE**. But I found, and I think you will find too, that the people administering your licensing exam are really nice, and really helpful. It's almost as if they know you are stressed out enough as it is. Most of them will regularly check on you, encourage you, and even tell you that you are going to pass *(not whether you actually did or not....but they will make you feel like you'll be ok)*. So from the time you arrive in the morning, be friendly and gracious with these people. It will make your day go better.

There seems to be a political component to the licensing exams. Much as I told you some places like Florida want to limit how many dentists come into their state to practice and compete with each other, it will seem like even these larger, more general licensing regions do the same thing. Call it a quota if you will, but when your exam is over, you will talk to students who had a disaster happen during the exam, and later you will find out they got a perfect score, while someone like yourself *(or like me....wink, wink)* was sure everything went perfectly and yet you received a failing score. These exams are expensive too as I previously mentioned and guess what....re-takes are also. Soooo.....I'll just leave you with this so I don't p*ss off any powers that be any more than I already have just by writing this book: sometimes the results don't make sense.

Alrighty then.... you will soon have your license to practice! Let's get away from dental school and tests and boards and exams finally, and start talking about getting your career going.

Chapter 7: Getting to Work in the Real World

Well, after four years of studying hard and dealing with all kinds of stress and bullcrap, you finally made it to the end and managed to graduate. You passed Part I and Part II of the National Board Exams. You took and passed a clinical licensing exam. You finished all of your requirements and received your dental degree *(possibly not in that order….my graduation was in May and I got out in July! Remember what I told you about your clinical requirements???)* So congratulations! Seriously, you have accomplished a lot….take a moment to pat yourself on the back as you have put yourself in a position to have a great life! *(Especially if you followed my advice about limiting your debt.)*

But you are just getting started now. You have to figure out where you go from here and how you want your career to unfold. It is exciting and daunting at the same time. Scary too, because you will soon realize you don't really know much about practicing dentistry!

Now, before I go into the various career paths you can take, I do want to talk briefly about post- graduate training. I am a general dentist who did a general practice residency (GPR) so I am going to focus on that, but your path will be similar even if you go into a specialty *(and you'll probably make more money)*.

If you are going into a specialty, obviously you have found a field that interests you and have to go through a residency to join that specialty. But if you are not going into a specialty, you could just go out and get a job doing dentistry, or even take the leap of buying or starting a practice *(but I wouldn't recommend either of these last two options yet....more on why in a bit)* or you can apply to a one year general practice residency. This is pretty much what it sounds like....you will spend a year doing general dentistry under supervision, though you will not be as supervised as a dental student...so no worries there! I'll go into a little more detail in a moment, but let me start by saying this:

DO YOURSELF A BIG FAVOR AND DO A GENERAL PRACTICE RESIDENCY!

In a general practice residency, you will gain a lot more experience doing all kinds of general dentistry procedures . You will be given a lot more leeway and freedom than you were in dental school....usually nobody is going to check your work unless you ask them too, and if and when they do they will not be critical of your work like they could be in dental school. No, the attending dentists in your residency are usually local dentists who are volunteering their time and often went through the program themselves. They will work with you and impart their knowledge and experience upon you to help you achieve a good outcome.

You will do a greater volume of procedures because the residency is usually operated as an actual practice or clinic, often for the underprivileged, so there are lots of patients.

And in doing more volume with experienced dentists, you will see many different ways of doing the same procedure. Also with the increased volume you will obviously become more skilled and your speed will go up. That's why they call it dental "practice" !

Now, most general practice residencies are "hospital-based". This means that your clinic can accommodate ill patients as well as patients of the hospital, and that you will most likely have an opportunity to take patients to the operating room to perform dentistry under general anesthesia. These may be ill patients who can't tolerate things like local anesthesia in clinic operatory, such as those with heart problems. They may be a combative learning disabled patient. They may just be someone who is scared and wants to be "put to sleep". They may even be an emergency such as a broken jaw who came in through the hospital emergency room and needs to see an attending oral surgeon, who will take you into the operating room with them to assist.

Regardless of the circumstances, it is **AWESOME** to work on people who are under general anesthesia. The anesthesiologist takes care of everything....you just do your dentistry. By the time you are done you will be thinking, "Man, doing open heart surgery under general anesthesia must be a hell of a lot easier than doing dentistry under local anesthesia!" *(Well, except for the high risk of your patient dying...)*

You may never practice dentistry like this again, but you can if you want to once you get out of your residency and settle somewhere, and it is a great service to offer your community as well as a potentially lucrative practice builder, as not a lot of general dentists do this for some reason.

Now, there is one minor drawback to being a resident in a hospital based general practice residency, and that is "on call" duty. This means that for a given period, usually a week, you will be the resident on call, or available 24/7, to the hospital, particularly the emergency room. It's actually not that bad, but you might get called in for an emergency at 2 am when you were sleeping, or for a consult for a physician at 5:15 pm when you were about to go home or out with friends. I don't really have much to say about it because there is nothing you can do about it, so suck it up and accept it as part of the residency. Sorry!

"Ok, Greg….isn't this chapter supposed to be about jobs in the real world? This residency thing sounds like school…."

Right, right...well, a specialty program might be like that, but guess what? A general practice residency position is a job, and you will probably get paid around $50,000 with benefits and vacation time. How does that sound? Pretty good compared to the last job you had doing what? Washing dishes at Olive Garden? *(Easy now- I was a dishwasher.)* That's not big money in dentistry terms, but it's still pretty good for a first job after dental school where you are learning a ton also, and believe me there are a lot of people out there who would love to make $50, 000 a year.

But I hear ya, my young and eager dentist friends…..

So as I said earlier, if you can, spend a year doing a general practice residency. You will be glad you did when you get your first "real" dental job, which we are going to talk about next…..

Back in the old days, the so-called "golden age of dentistry" when you could graduate without soul-crushing debt and insurance wasn't a big factor in the industry, many new dentists could simply "hang a shingle" with their name on it and start a new practice, grow it, live a prosperous life and retire wealthy.

This era probably ended sometime in the 1980's, and with the rising cost of becoming a dentist as well as the growing influence of insurance and their crappy fee schedules, it is most likely gone for good. And because of this, the entire industry has changed and there are different ways of getting started. But fear not. With the right decisions and timing you can still end up in the same place as the dentists from that bygone era!

Your options for employment as a new dentist are:

1. **An associateship (working for someone established in private practice)**

2. **Corporate dentistry (working for a "dental service organization" such as Aspen Dental or Heartland Dental among others)**

3. **Working for the government as a civilian (for example at a Veteran's Administration (VA) Hospital or dental clinic or as a civilian on a military base)**

4. **Working for the government as an officer in the military, which was touched on earlier in this book**

5. **Starting your own dental practice "from scratch"**

6. **Buying an established dental practice**

So let's discuss these options.

Associateship

The majority of new dentists, whether right out of school or a general practice residency, start off working as an associate in an established dental practice that either needs help because it is busy or the practice's owner is looking to slow down and possibly retire.

Associateships can go a lot of ways and rather than counsel you in detail on what to look for I suggest you do some research into what to look for as there are tons of articles online about this. However I will boil it down to a few key points.

1. **Pay:** generally you will get a daily rate (probably $400-500/ day) as a base and a percentage of either your production or collections, somewhere in the 30-35% range. Sometimes your lab expenses (such as getting crowns made) are deducted from this percentage. Try to get it as a percentage of your production, as collection is usually lower because insurance doesn't pay your full fee, or the patient simply didn't pay and/or the front desk failed to collect the money!

2. **Procedures:** Sure, the dentist hiring you doesn't know you that well so obviously he's not going to give you some huge case right away, but make sure you're not just going to be doing hygiene checks and fillings all day. How are you going to make any of the money we talked about above? Plus, it will get boring, and you want to get more experienced doing all kinds of procedures!

3. **The owner (ie your boss):** There are all kinds of dentists out there. I already ranted about the crazy ones running most dental schools. Your boss could be like that and make working in his/her office suck. Dentists like this are usually control freaks and think their office is something special and that they are the best dentists in the world. They will nitpick over what you do, how you do it, and in the end make you feel like you suck as a dentist. Nevermind that you don't have a lot of experience and want to learn from them. These types will also find a way to rip you off with your pay. So if you get this vibe from a potential boss, or actually work for someone like this, look elsewhere....you want someone like my old boss when I was an associate.....someone cool! Dentists like this are good practitioners and have nice, established offices, but they are relaxed. They know you are new and inexperienced, and want to show you how to practice dentistry in the real world. If you work for a really cool dentist they will even teach you about the business side of dentistry. They are really only looking for someone decent to to come in and lighten their workload so they can have more leisure time and think about retiring.....which leads to my next point.

4. **Future plans:** As I just said, hopefully you have a great boss who is contemplating retirement. If this is the case and you are working in a nice, well-run and productive office, you may have hit the career jackpot! That is, you work there for a year or two, learn how the place runs, then take over the office in a relatively seamless

transition. As an alternative, if your boss isn't planning on retiring for a while, you may be able to become a partner in the practice, where you "buy in" to the practice so you are a co-owner. I'll discuss ownership options in more detail shortly.

Corporate Dentistry

The last two decades have seen the rise of the so-called "corporate" dental practices. These are basically large companies that operate multiple dental office all over the place. An example is Aspen Dental. They are based out of Syracuse, New York and started in the late 1990's with less than twenty offices. Today there are over five hundred Aspen Dental practices all over the United States.

Businesses like this are run as very efficient, profit-driven organizations. They are frequently run by business people who are not dentists. A lot of the time they are "owned" by large, private equity investment companies, which basically invest wealthy people's money in businesses that they think will grow rapidly, increasing in value and thus allowing them to "cash out" later with significant profits.

Corporate groups like this can be a great place for new dentists to start their careers. However there are pros and cons to working for these outfits. I know because I worked for one for a while. Now keep in mind that although the various corporate dental companies are similar, they of course do have differences. So if you are looking into working for one, use what I am about tell you as a guideline, and ask lots of questions before you sign on, and re-visit these issues while you are working there. Frequently.

Did you see that last word? Frequently. Be sure to re-visit how things are going for you **FREQUENTLY** if you find yourself working for one of these organizations. Make sure you are happy! You will understand shortly. Ok....here we go...

Pros of working in corporate dentistry:

1. **A guaranteed job:** Most corporate dental companies are desperate for new associates *(you'll see why in the "cons"....)*. Unless you have some serious issues and/or make a terrible impression, you'll get hired. These companies may even try to recruit you before you graduate or finish a residency.

2. **Money:** The pay packages these companies offer are usually pretty enticing, especially if you are coming right out of school or a residency. Your base salary should be at least $100,000-$150,000, and there are bonus incentives that frequently push income to the $250,000-$300,000 range. I know......wow, right? Again, you'll see some of the cons below. In addition to generous pay packages, you will also get a benefit package that includes your health insurance, vacation and sick time, et cetera. Usually these companies also take care of your malpractice insurance premiums.

3. **Skill development:** I know the money sounds great, but the biggest benefit a new dentist will get working for a corporate outfit is skill and speed development. You will see **A TON** of patients and do **A TON** of procedures. **ALL KINDS OF PROCEDURES**. Your skill and speed will naturally increase with each day, week, month and year you spend there. *(Notice*

the bold print.....again, you'll read the cons below in a minute.)

4. **You might make a boatload of money:** Remember above when I said these companies might be run by business people who aren't dentists? Yeeeeahhh that's not really allowed in a lot of states. Generally a dental office has to be run by a dentist. So what a lot of these companies have done is "sell" these practices to the dentists that work in them, or in some cases they'll "sell" a group of practices in a particular region to one of their dentists. Sometimes these dentists will sell partnerships to their associates who work in their offices if they do in fact own multiple offices. Now, the original corporate dental company, who used to "own" the practices, will call themselves a "dental service organization", or DSO. They will charge the "owner" dentists they "sold" the practices to a consultation fee to help run the business side of things *(weird how it is always somewhere around 45-55% of revenues....but it's not a partnership or anything, right? Wink wink....).* You'll understand why I'm using quotes when you, again, read the "cons" in a minute. But here's the main point- these places are in business to make money, and they make a lot of it. If you own the practice and the corporate side is doing what they went into business to do anyway, you will get a bigger chunk than if you just work there. Like, $250,000+. Per office. With associates of yours doing the work in the offices you're not at. Whoaaaa, right? So, do the math if you "own" three, four or five offices. Do you see what I'm talking about?

Ok so those were some of the "pros" of working in corporate dentistry. Now let's look at some of the pitfalls of working in this setting.

Cons of working in corporate dentistry:

1. **The almighty dollar rules:** No matter what catch-line or mission statement or ad campaign any of these companies are running, always remember that these are businesses that exist to make money and profits first and foremost. Remember that and keep reading....

2. **You will work your butt off:** In the name of making money, these types of offices want the schedule maximized. Of course in any office you don't want to be sitting around, but in a private office on a busy day between yourself **and** hygiene you might see twenty to thirty patients a day whereas in a corporate setting you could see forty **just on your own**. And the better you handle it, the more they will stuff your schedule. You will be exhausted and worn out at the end of each day, week, month....

3. **Referring is frowned upon:** Again, in the name of making money, most corporate offices want to keep as much of the work "in-house" as possible, so they will prefer that you don't refer stuff such as extractions and root canals to specialists. Now most of these places won't force you to do stuff, but you will feel pressure and it will be brought up to you, probably initially at the suggestion of people who don't know much about dentistry. Read on.....

4. **The corporate influence:** As I said earlier, most of these companies are run by non-dental

business people. There have been some entrepreneurial dentists who have started some of these outfits, but by the time they get big there are usually plenty of non-dentist executives helping to run things. And on a more local level they usually have district and regional managers as well as individual office managers who before working there, worked for companies like Heinz or some retailer like Macy's. Now because many of these companies have come under scrutiny for having these non-dentist people influence clinical decisions, which is a big no-no, they usually insist that all clinical decisions are made by the dentists exclusively. Go ahead and check their websites and the small print in their ads. But make no mistake....the suits are watching and making sure things are done a certain way and that profits are being made. Usually this is done by working with the "owner" dentist, who wants to maximize profits anyway. So after the "owner" has a meeting with the executives, THEY will be the one who, as the "owner", will tell you, the associate, how you "should" be doing things. And basically, over time, if in their eyes, you aren't productive and making the office and the company enough money, you will be fired and replaced by one of the many people applying to work there.

5. **The stigma of working in corporate dentistry:** Within the profession, corporate dentistry is generally looked at with a skeptical eye, generally because of their reputation for being primarily profit driven and doing things such as aggressively treatment planning, seeing too many patients, and doing shoddy work.

Personally I think it comes down to the individual doctor and their ethical standards, but unfortunately you will still be seen as one of the "bad doctors who works for the terrible corporate dental organization", and this kind of makes the meet and greets at dental meetings a little awkward. However, corporate dentistry is probably here to stay, and because of changes in the industry with costs and insurance and new dentists with a lot of debt, it probably has its place. But it does scare the so-called "old guard".

6. **If you become an "owner", you are not a true owner:** Did you notice above my use of quotes whenever I used the word "owner"? You did? Great....because when you own a dental practice you control everything, except maybe the space you work in because you might lease it. In the corporate setting, you are really more of a partner. Think about it....if the corporation found the space, built the office, and paid for all the equipment, do you think as the "owner" you could find another space and move there, taking everything with you? No. No more so than the owner of a Subway sandwich shop could. You are a partner with the corporation, and it will be legally set up in such a way so as to separate the corporation from the clinical side of things, and you will be designated the "owner" who controls the clinical side. Now, this set-up generally works great if you can accept its limitations.....you can make a lot of money, but you will never have the 100% autonomy that true ownership provides.

Working for the Government as a Civilian

When I first got out of my residency, I worked on a Native American Reservation . There were some levels of separation, but basically I was working for US Government. There are other government jobs such as working at a Veteran's Administration Hospital or working as a civilian on a military base. These can be great jobs to get your feet wet, as well as possibly build a career.

Some **pros** of this type of job:

1. You **just show up and do the work**. No worries about getting patients, production, collection, insurance, or basically running the place.

2. Usually you get **nice facilities and equipment**, and if you need something, there is a budget but usually the government will get it for you. *(If they'll buy an $800 toilet seat, they'll buy you a new handpiece...I mean drill).*

3. **Steady pay**. Again, no worries about production and collection.

4. **Great benefits**. You should get a nice package including health insurance, retirement, paid vacation and sick time, as a well as some other cool perks depending on your situation, such as access to government facilities like a gym if you work on a base.

5. Your job could lead to a **steady, long term career**.

Now, some **cons** of working for the government:

1. The **pay is never that great** compared to what you will make working in private practice or in

corporate dentistry, unless you are there for years and work your way into some high paying *(ie government bloat)* administrative job.

2. It can be **hard to stay motivated** when you know you will get paid the same whether you do a lot of dentistry or not a lot of dentistry.

3. If you are in a situation where the **patients** are getting the work you do for free via the government, you will get annoyed at how this causes them to not really care about taking care of their teeth or not showing up for their appointments. *("It's free so who cares!"....Get used to that.)*

4. **Bureaucracy**. This is the government of course. You will have superiors you'll have to answer to.

5. Once again, you may get a **nagging feeling** of dissatisfaction from not being independent like many of your colleagues.

Working for the Government as an Officer in the Military

I touched on this earlier when I talked about paying for dental school, but I personally was never in the military, so I am not going to go into great detail here. Many of the benefits and disadvantages of this career path are similar to working for the government as a civilian *(the biggest difference being the possibility of being deployed to a war zone....kind of a big deal....).* If you have an obligation to the military because of any help they gave you getting your education, you will have plenty of exposure and time to consider this career path anyway, right?

Your Own Private Practice

The next two things I am going to talk about are starting your own practice or buying someone else's practice.

Now, there are plenty of resources out there about practice ownership and all details about running your own practice, so I am not going to go into all those details here.

Just keep in mind that whichever way you go, owning your own practice is probably the best way to achieve personal and professional success. You will most likely earn more than in any other setting, and more importantly, you will get to keep more of what you work for. Not only because you are the owner but also because there are a lot of sweet tax benefits from owning your own business. As you grow and achieve success you will have a tremendous feeling of satisfaction. Thus, this is the goal and path of most dentists. If you feel this is the way you want to go, you should go for it as soon as you think you are ready *(but not before then or it could be a disaster!)*

Starting a Dental Practice "from Scratch"

It's probably pretty obvious from what I said earlier that owning your own dental practice is usually goal of most dentists. Starting your own practice from nothing is the most difficult way to do this, because of the inherent risks and time it takes to develop into a successful business. However it can also be the most rewarding and satisfying, because it is all yours- you came up with the idea, implemented it, made it happen and made it successful.

If you are a relatively new dentist, I don't recommend this at this point in your career. However if you do have some experience, and you don't have too many responsibilities besides yourself *(like a family to feed)*, and you like the excitement of doing your own thing, then go for it!

Buying an Established Dental Practice

I mentioned above that if you are a new dentist, I don't recommend starting your own practice. However, if you are experienced and have a family **and** financial responsibilities, I don't recommend it either.

But...owning your own practice is what you want.....so what should you do?

Buy someone else's established practice!

I know starting your own practice from scratch sounds like the most exciting way to have your own practice, and it may be. If you are in the right situation, it may be the right decision for you, but buying an established practice from a retiring dentist is **BY FAR** the best way to get to where you want to be both professionally and personally.

How do I know???

I know because that's where I am now, and I waited too long to get here!

Let me list some pros and cons *(I know...again)* of buying an existing dental practice:

Pros:

1. **You are buying an existing patient base and income stream.** This is business, and you are buying something valuable, so get over the whole being a dentist thing and realize you are taking over a business just like in any other industry. You are still going to do dentistry *(obviously)*, but what you are buying will provide you income and allow you to live life hopefully the way you want to. If you start your own practice from nothing, it will take you a couple of years at least to get to where you will be the day you take over an established practice.

2. **An established practice basically runs itself**. That is, along with the long term staff who you will want to keep. Yes you can make changes and tweak things once you are the owner, but wait a little while to do that. The existing patients that you want to stay with you will appreciate this.

3. **It is easier to get a bank loan to buy an established practice.** Financing dental practice acquisitions is usually a slam dunk for lenders. When was the last time you heard of a dental practice going out of business? Especially one that has already been around for twenty or thirty years?

4. **There are none, or at least fewer, of the headaches of trying to start a practice from scratch.** Coordinating things such as finding and leasing a space, getting financed,

overseeing construction, getting permits, hiring staff, getting patients in the door.....there is way more to worry about than with taking over an existing practice.

Cons:

1. **It takes a while for the practice to become "yours"**. Remember, you are buying an existing business that has been operating without **you** for a long time. People are used to the way things have been. Patients are used to the existing staff, especially the doctor! But be patient. Set your ego aside. Settle in, don't be in a rush to "make it yours", and after not too long, it will be yours, and staff and patients will recognize this.

2. **You may not like all the staff.** Sort of like above....give it a little time before you make changes *(unless there is a big problem).*

3. **You may have to deal with some of the previous owner's work that you don't like..or worse.** Dealing with remakes and failures of old work is something that your attorney should address in your purchase agreement.

4. **The office may take insurance you don't like.** Again, give it some time, analyze things, then later you can make changes.

These are the really big things that kind of suck when you take over someone's practice. I didn't mention things like crappy, old equipment or things you don't like about the office space like the decor because those are things you should use to negotiate the selling price, plus you can and probably will get your own equipment and change the look of **YOUR** office in time.

Regardless of the career path you follow, there are two things you should remember:

1. **Learn from every experience you have**. Doing so has enabled me to get to the experience to feel qualified *(somewhat)* to write this book!

2. **Don't waste time being unhappy!** There are too many ways for you to work and practice dentistry. For myself, I probably spent too long in corporate dentistry because I was making crazy money. I'm much happier with the lifestyle private practice affords me *(and come on....I'm a dentist and still do pretty well compared to most people)*.

Wow....that last bit there sounded like I'm giving away some so-called "pearls of wisdom". Maybe I'm almost done writing this book.

That gives me an idea for the last chapter........

Chapter 8: Miscellaneous Stuff ...

That Didn't Really Fit Into the Other Chapters in This Book Because It Would Have Made Them Too Long and Ponderous Like the Title of this Chapter

So I want to say a few things before I wrap this book up, things that I've learned or come to realize over the course of my career. If you are starting out, keep these things in mind as you move forward. If you are an established dentist, as with this book, consider what I am saying....you may agree or disagree, but I at least hope to give you another perspective. Here we go in no particular order....just random thoughts.

1. **Always put your patients first.** Your patients are your customers, and just like in every other business, the customer is always right *(even when they aren't)*. Yeah, yeah....you're a doctor blah blah blah.....look, if you want to be successful, give your patients what they want, within clinical reason. If **you** don't, someone else will.

2. **Don't worry about perfection.** Your brutal dental school instructors may have left you with an inferiority complex. Guess what? Nobody is checking your work in the real world. As long as you remove the decay, and seal the margins,

nobody is going to give you a problem if the anatomy in a filling on tooth #15 isn't lifelike!

3. **But don't take shortcuts.** This goes hand in hand with 1 and 2 above. You always have to do right by your patient. Don't do a crappy job and if there is a problem, don't ignore it- discuss it with your patient. They will appreciate your honesty, and most importantly, they will trust you.

4. **Don't ignore your state's regulations.** I haven't had too much trouble with this, but I have had to scramble a few times to get all my continuing education   completed when I had three years to do it. The state can shut you down or worse, so don't mess around with this!

5. **Prescription writing is a privilege.** Again, relating to number 4, don't mess around with this. Don't prescribe out of your scope of practice for your friend's urinary tract infection. And only prescribe narcotics as absolutely needed.

6. **Have a good accountant and attorney.** You'll need an accountant to help you manage your taxes, and it's always good to have an attorney who knows you who can help you when trouble comes up, or if you just need some questions answered.

7. **Find a good chiropractor.** Practicing dentistry is very physical, and can wreak havoc on your neck, back, and shoulders. A chiropractor can work wonders....I know first hand. In addition to this, be sure to take care of your overall health in general!

8. **Don't live beyond your means.** You went through a lot to become a dentist. You probably make a good living. It's tempting to get that BMW and a big "doctor's house". Don't do it if you really can't afford it!

9. **Put money away.** Instead of paying a fat mortgage or making that Mercedes payment, start saving for retirement, and building some savings in case of an emergency. Take advantage of the miracle that is compound interest.

10. **Pay off your debts.** Hopefully you took my earlier advice and aren't hugely indebted, but work on paying off those student loans if you have any, or your practice loan if you have one.

11. **Own your own practice as soon into your career as you can.** I know I touched on this earlier, and there are many career paths you can take, but if you think this is what you ultimately want to do, do it as soon as you think you can handle it.

12. **When you have a practice, try to own the building you are in also.** Did you used to live in apartment? Did you get sick of throwing money away on rent instead of building equity? You did? Ok then.....same thing. Plus there are lots of tax benefits and you will thank me *(or at least hopefully remember this book)* when you are ready to retire.

13. **Patients don't care about granite countertops.** In other words don't waste money on stuff like this, or the latest and greatest technology for that matter. Patients don't care.

14. **All that patients really care about is that you fix their teeth without hurting or scaring them, in a safe and clean environment.** See 13 above. Don't let your ego hurt your business. Think like a plumber or carpenter, not a dentist. Which reminds me......

15. **Speak English.** Not literally, but spare your patients all the dental terminology. It just confuses and intimidates them, and lessens their likelihood to accept treatment.

16. **Don't do stuff you don't like just for money.** Unless it's easy, stay away from big dollar procedures you don't like to do. Otherwise you will eventually start to hate being a dentist.

17. **Don't feel inferior when you read dental journals and magazines.** This one can creep up on you. You'll read about all the millionaire dentists doing full arch implants using their cone beam x-ray machine in their practice they opened six months ago. Don't believe all the hype. Do the best you can at what you like to do and that is good enough if you are happy.

18. **Sometimes the old stuff is the best stuff.** Like with technology, try not to get to caught up in every new product and "clinical breakthrough" you see. There are a lot of dentists out there trying to invent something to get themselves out of practicing dentistry.....get what I'm saying? My rule is if it's been being used for five or more years I **might** try it, but do I really need it?

19. **Learn to extract teeth and make dentures.** These can be really easy and really lucrative

procedures. Surprisingly, not a lot of general dentists pull teeth!

20. **Leave work at work.** You might love dentistry, but a lot of dentists seem to let it be like a hobby for them. That's fine, and if you love it that much great, but there's nothing wrong with saying it's a tough job and you really don't want to think about it outside of work. One of the things I absolutely hate about dental meetings is that in conversation, some dentists only want to talk about clinical stuff!

21. **Marry the RIGHT person.** You will have an opportunity for a great life. Of course it will be better if you can share it with someone. You want to be on the same page with that person in terms of how you both want to live your lives together, as a team. If you do, you will achieve even more success and satisfaction. If you don't, even if you reset, it could result in a setback that will never allow you to reach your full potential.

22. **If you find that person, do what you can not to lose them.** On the flip side, if they aren't the right person, don't be afraid to let them go.

23. **There is nothing more important or precious than children.** Whether they are yours or someone else's. And if they are yours, make every sacrifice you have to in order to be the best parent you can be to them.

24. **Take vacations and enjoy life with your family.** Dentistry will still be there when you get back!

25. Get a dog. Dogs are awesome. *(I'm partial...but I'm sure this is true for all pets.)*

Well, it looks like I've just about covered everything I wanted to as I was thinking about what I wanted to put in this book. Like I said at the beginning, I wanted this book to really help those who have just barely started their journey to becoming a dentist, but I also wanted it to be a decent read for really any dentist at any point in their career. I'm sure there will be plenty of people out there who will read this and think I'm an idiot *(I see you dental school administrators and hardcore dentists whose lives revolve around your careers...)* but I bet there will be plenty of practicing dentists like me who will say, "This guy Greg really nailed it.....I wish this book was around when I was starting out!" Hopefully some of the people thinking about a career in dentistry or just starting out in dental school will read this and join the ones that like the book.

Regardless, whether you liked it or hated it, whether you like me or think I'm a moron, thank you for taking the time to read this book. I truly do appreciate it! No matter where you are in your dental career, I wish you health, happiness and good fortune. Remember, as I said at the beginning of this book....

DENTISTRY ISN'T BRAIN SURGERY....SO DON'T GET SO STRESSED OUT!

www.ingramcontent.com/pod-product-compliance
Lightning Source LLC
Chambersburg PA
CBHW061220180526
45170CB00003B/1085